IRRITABLE BOWEL SYNDROME (IBS) DIET COOKBOOK

Delicious Low-Fodmap Recipes, And Gut-Friendly Foods For Reversing Symptoms, Reducing Bloating, Improving Digestive Health And More

DR. AMARI VALERIE

TABLE OF CONTENTS

BONUS:

7 days meal plan recipes, ingredients, and detailed preparatory guidelines for Irritable bowel syndrome (IBS)

7 Desserts procedural recipes for Irritable bowel syndrome (IBS) and guidelines

7 Smoothies procedural recipes for Irritable bowel syndrome (IBS) and guidelines

DISCLAIMER

The information provided in this book, is for educational and informational purposes only and is not intended as medical advice. The content is not a substitute for professional medical advice, diagnosis, or treatment. Always seek the advice of your physician or other qualified health provider with any questions you may have regarding a medical condition. Never disregard professional medical advice or delay in seeking it because of something you have read in this book.

The dietary suggestions and recipes in this book are based on general guidelines and may not be suitable for everyone. Individual responses to foods can vary, and it is important to consult with a healthcare professional before making any significant changes to your diet.

The author and publisher of this book do not claim to cure or treat any medical condition. The information provided is based on research and personal experience and is intended to help readers make informed decisions about their diet and health.

Furthermore, I the author do not endorse any specific products, brands, treatments, or services that may be mentioned in this book. Any references to products, services, websites, or organizations are provided for informational purposes only and do not constitute an endorsement or recommendation by the author. The inclusion of such references does not imply any association, sponsorship, or affiliation between the author and the referenced entities.

The recipes and dietary suggestions in this book are designed to be safe and healthful. However, readers should use their own discretion and consult with a healthcare professional when necessary, especially if they have allergies, sensitivities, or other dietary restrictions.

By using this book, you acknowledge and agree that the author and publisher shall not be held liable for any loss or damage, including but not limited to special, incidental, consequential, or other damages, resulting from the use of the information and recipes contained in this book.

ABOUT THIS BOOK

For individuals who are interested in comprehending and managing this prevalent gastrointestinal disorder, the publication "Irritable Bowel Syndrome (IBS)" is an indispensable resource.

The introduction establishes the context by emphasizing the importance of IBS and the profound influence it can have on daily life. Subsequently, a comprehensive explanation of the fundamentals and symptoms of IBS is provided, which includes a precise definition, the different varieties, and the condition's widespread prevalence. It also underscores the critical role of diet in the management of IBS symptoms, thereby establishing the foundation for more in-depth discussions on dietary interventions.

The Low-FODMAP diet is thoroughly examined, commencing with an explanation of FODMAPs and their role in IBS. This book delineates the advantages of adhering to a low-FODMAP diet, including an enhanced quality of life and diminished symptoms. Practical advice regarding which foods to avoid and which to incorporate, as well as a comprehensive guide to the various phases of the diet, will be provided to readers.

Additionally, the fundamentals of nutrition for digestive health are thoroughly addressed. This book delves into the significance of a well-balanced diet and the precise function of fiber in the preservation of digestive health. It emphasizes the importance of adequate hydration and the advantages of probiotics and prebiotics in the development of a healthy intestine. The following tips are provided to assist readers in making informed dietary choices by identifying and avoiding trigger foods.

Insights into the potential cure of IBS, the typical duration for the Low-FODMAP diet to take effect, and the steps to take if symptoms do not improve are provided in this book, which also addresses common concerns and frequently asked questions. Practical guidance is provided for effectively managing IBS flare-ups and adhering to a low-FODMAP diet while dining out.

This book offers comprehensive guidance on meal planning, grocery purchasing, and meal preparation for individuals who are just beginning their IBS diet voyage. Readers are adequately prepared to initiate their dietary modifications by following guidelines for interpreting food labels and establishing achievable objectives.

The thorough chapters on diet and recipes are particularly beneficial. Readers will acquire knowledge regarding the significance of personalized dietary plans, the influence of diet on IBS symptoms, and the advantages of maintaining a food diary. The comparison between low-FODMAP and High-FODMAP foods and the explanation of FODMAPs are both informative. This book is a practical guide for daily living, featuring practical sections on the creation of a Low-FODMAP pantry and delectable, easy-to-follow recipes for breakfast, lunch, supper, snacking, and desserts.

In addition to recipes, this book contains seven-day meal plans, dessert recipes, and smoothie recipes, each of which includes comprehensive preparatory instructions. This methodical approach facilitates the seamless integration of the Low-FODMAP diet into the lives of readers.

Lastly, this book offers strategies for nutrition planning and advice for achieving long-term success. Strategies for weekly meal planning, bulk cookery, and managing social situations and dining out are addressed to guarantee that readers can sustain their digestive health over the long term. This book is a comprehensive and practical guide for individuals with IBS, providing the knowledge and tools necessary to effectively manage the condition. It is a standout.

CHAPTER ONE

Basics And Symptoms Of IBS: An Overview

Irritable bowel syndrome (IBS) is a chronic gastrointestinal disorder that is distinguished by diarrhea, constipation, or a combination of the two, as well as abdominal discomfort and inflammation. Common symptoms include abdominal pain, discomfort, flatulence, and diarrhea or constipation, which are frequently precipitated by specific foods or stress.

IBS is classified into three primary categories based on the predominant symptoms: IBS-D (diarrhea-predominant), IBS-C (constipation-predominant), and IBS-M (mixt). This condition has a substantial impact on daily life by causing distress and impeding regular activities. Dietary modifications are frequently necessary to alleviate symptoms and enhance quality of life to effectively manage IBS.

IBS Definition

Irritable intestine Syndrome (IBS) is a functional gastrointestinal disorder that lacks a recognized organic cause. Despite its appearance, the intestine does not function normally. It is a prevalent condition that impacts the large intestine and is diagnosed by observing symptoms such as recurrent abdominal pain that is associated with bowel movements and changes in feces frequency or form.

IBS is a chronic condition that necessitates long-term management through lifestyle and dietary modifications to alleviate symptoms and improve overall digestive health.

Common Symptoms

Abdominal pain or discomfort, bloating, gas, and changes in bowel patterns, such as diarrhea, constipation, or an alternation between the two, are among the most prevalent symptoms of IBS. These symptoms frequently exhibit fluctuations in intensity and may be precipitated by hormonal fluctuations, tension, or specific substances. For example, certain individuals may experience symptoms that are exacerbated by the consumption of dairy, fattening foods, or caffeine. Maintaining a symptom diary to monitor food intake and symptoms can assist in the identification and prevention of triggers, thereby facilitating the management of IBS.

Different Types Of IBS

Each variety of IBS is classified by the predominant bowel habit. There are three primary categories of IBS.

Frequent, unstable movements and urgency are the hallmarks of IBS-D (diarrhea-predominant). Infrequent, firm stools and difficulty passing stools are symptoms of IBS-C (constipation-predominant). IBS-M (mixed) encompasses both diarrhea and constipation.

It is essential to comprehend the specific type of IBS you have, as this enables the customization of dietary and treatment regimens to address the distinctive symptoms associated with each type, thereby ensuring the more effective management of the condition.

Impact On Daily Life And Prevalence

IBS is estimated to affect 10-15% of the global population, with a higher prevalence in women than in males. The condition can have a substantial impact on daily life by causing persistent distress, which can result in delayed work or social activities and a reduced quality of life.

Because of the unpredictable nature of their symptoms, individuals with IBS frequently experience anxiety and depression. These impacts can be mitigated and overall well-being can be enhanced through effective management through diet, stress reduction, and medical intervention.

The Significance Of Diet In The Management Of IBS

The management of IBS symptoms is significantly influenced by the diet. Symptoms may be precipitated by specific substances, while others may mitigate them. For instance, there is evidence that a limited FODMAP diet is beneficial for numerous individuals with IBS, as it reduces the absorption of specific carbohydrates that are inadequately absorbed in the intestine.

Limiting the consumption of foods such as garlic, shallots, and wheat is recommended while incorporating soluble fiber from sources such as oats and specific fruits can facilitate digestion. The quality of life and symptom management can be substantially enhanced by collaborating with a dietitian to develop a personalized dietary plan.

CHAPTER TWO

An Overview Of The Low-FODMAP Diet

The Low-FODMAP diet is a specialized dietary regimen that is intended to assist in the management of symptoms associated with irritable bowel syndrome (IBS).

It entails the reduction of foods that are high in fermentable oligosaccharides, disaccharides, monosaccharides, and polyols (FODMAPs), which can cause abdominal pain, flatulence, and bloating.

The diet is typically implemented in three phases: elimination, reintroduction, and personalization. The objective is to identify and restrict specific FODMAPs that induce symptoms in individuals.

What are FODMAPs?

FODMAPs are sugar alcohols and short-chain carbohydrates that are present in a variety of foods. However, they are not well assimilated in the small intestine. fructose (found in fruits and honey), lactose (found in dairy products), fructans (found in wheat, garlic, and scallions), Galatians (found in legumes and lentils), and polyols (found in certain fruits and artificial sweeteners) are among them. In individuals with IBS, symptoms such as diarrhea, flatulence, and bloating may result from the fermentation of these compounds in the intestines.

Advantages Of A Low-FODMAP Diet For IBS

The severity and frequency of IBS symptoms can be significantly reduced by implementing a low-FODMAP diet. Bloating, flatulence, abdominal pain, and irregular bowel movements are alleviated by numerous individuals. Individuals can develop a more personalized and effective approach to managing their IBS by systematically eliminating and reintroducing FODMAPs, which enables them to identify their specific triggers.

Foods To Avoid

It is essential to refrain from consuming high-FODMAP foods that may exacerbate symptoms of IBS when adhering to a low-FODMAP diet.

The following are common culprits: certain fruits (such as apples, pears, and mangoes), vegetables (such as garlic, onions, and cauliflower), dairy products containing lactose (such as milk and soft cheeses), legumes (such as beans and lentils), and specific cereals (such as wheat and rye). Furthermore, it is advisable to refrain from consuming artificial sweeteners, such as sorbitol and mannitol.

Foods That Are Safe To Consume

There are numerous secure foods to consume while adhering to a low-FODMAP diet. These consist of low-FODMAP fruits, such as strawberries, blueberries, and oranges; vegetables, such as carrots, spinach, and bell peppers; lactose-free dairy alternatives, such as almond milk and firm cheeses; cereals, such as rice, quinoa, and gluten-free bread; and proteins, such as chicken, beef, and tofu. These foods contribute to the preservation of a well-balanced diet while simultaneously alleviating symptoms of IBS.

Phases Of The Low-FODMAP Diet

The low-FODMAP diet is implemented in three distinct phases. Elimination is the initial phase, which entails the abstinence from all high-FODMAP substances for a period of 4-6 weeks to alleviate symptoms.

The second phase, reintroduction, entails the progressive reintroduction of high-FODMAP foods one at a time to determine which specific foods induce symptoms. In the final phase, personalization, a long-term eating plan is developed that restricts only the identified trigger foods while ensuring a balanced and varied diet.

CHAPTER THREE

Digestive Health Nutritional Fundamentals

It is essential to consume a well-balanced diet that includes a variety of nutrients, including proteins, lipids, carbohydrates, vitamins, and minerals, to preserve digestive health.

To guarantee that your body receives the necessary nutrients, consume a diverse array of fruits, vegetables, lean proteins (including chicken, fish, and legumes), and whole cereals.

For instance, a nutritious meal might consist of grilled salmon, quinoa, and a side of steamed asparagus. This diversity is beneficial for the overall health of the intestines and can alleviate the symptoms of IBS.

The Function Of Fiber In The Digestive Process

Fiber is essential for the regulation of gastrointestinal movements and the enhancement of assimilation. Soluble fiber, which is present in foods such as oats, apples, and vegetables, aids in the softening of stool, whereas insoluble fiber, which is present in whole grains and legumes, contributes volume to the stool. To facilitate practical integration, you could commence your day with a bowl of oatmeal that is garnished with hazelnuts and sliced pears. Bloating and discomfort that are commonly associated with IBS can be prevented by gradually increasing fiber intake.

The Influence Of Hydration On Gut Health

Maintaining proper hydration is crucial for digestive health, as water facilitates the digestion of food and the absorption of nutrients. It is recommended that you consume a minimum of eight glasses of water per day, with an additional eight glasses if you are physically active. To guarantee consistent hydration, it is recommended that you carry a reusable water container and consume portions throughout the day. Proper hydration is essential for the seamless passage of food through the digestive tract and the prevention of constipation.

Prebiotics And Probiotics

Fermented foods, including yogurt, kefir, and sauerkraut, contain probiotics, which are beneficial bacteria that aid in the preservation of intestinal flora homeostasis. These beneficial microbes are nourished by prebiotics, which are present in foods such as scallions, bananas, and garlic. A practicable method of incorporating these into your diet is to consume a serving of Greek yogurt with a banana for breakfast. This combination is essential for the management of IBS symptoms, as it promotes a healthy intestinal microbiome.

Identifying And Avoiding Trigger Foods

The key to managing IBS is the identification and avoidance of trigger foods. Dairy, gluten, caffeine, and specific high-FODMAP foods, such as scallions and legumes, are frequently identified as triggers.

Maintain a food diary to monitor your diet and document any symptoms that may develop. For example, if you experience discomfort after consuming bread, consider substituting it with a gluten-free alternative.

This personalized method aids in the identification and elimination of foods that exacerbate symptoms of IBS.

CHAPTER FOUR

Frequently Asked Questions And Common Concerns

It is not uncommon to have queries and concerns when managing IBS. For example, it is crucial to comprehend food triggers, maintain nutritional adequacy, and balance dietary restrictions.

Furthermore, it can be difficult to differentiate between IBS and other gastrointestinal conditions, manage unpredictable symptoms, and navigate social situations. Consult a healthcare professional for personalized guidance at all times.

Is It Possible To Cure IBS?

IBS cannot be cured; however, it can be effectively managed through lifestyle modifications, dietary adjustments, and, in some cases, medication.

Symptoms can be substantially alleviated by increasing fiber intake, avoiding known trigger foods, and implementing a low-FODMAP diet. Furthermore, IBS symptoms may be alleviated through stress management strategies such as meditation, yoga, and consistent physical activity.

How Long Does It Take For The Low-FODMAP Diet To Become Effective?

It typically takes approximately 4-6 weeks for the Low-FODMAP diet to produce substantial improvements. It entails an elimination phase, during which high-FODMAP foods are eliminated from the diet, and a reintroduction phase that is designed to identify specific triggers.

Under the supervision of a dietitian, it is essential to maintain a food diary during this period to monitor symptoms and responses to various foods.

If the Low-FODMAP diet fails to alleviate symptoms, it may be beneficial to consult with a healthcare professional regarding the possibility of reassessing one's diet and lifestyle. They may recommend alternative dietary strategies, prescribe medications to manage symptoms, or suggest additional testing for other conditions. Some individuals may also benefit from psychological therapies, such as cognitive behavioral therapy (CBT).

How Can One Navigate Dining Out While Adhering To A Low-FODMAP Diet?

Careful preparation is necessary when dining out on a low-FODMAP diet. In advance, review restaurant menus, select straightforward dishes such as grilled meat or seafood with vegetables, and refrain from consuming high-FODMAP ingredients such as garlic and shallots. Inform the restaurant personnel of your dietary restrictions and do not hesitate to inquire about the preparation of the dishes. It can also be beneficial to bring a list of safe dishes or FODMAP-friendly applications.

Managing Flare-Ups Of IBS

The management of IBS flare-ups entails the identification and avoidance of triggers, the maintenance of a balanced diet, and the utilization of relaxation techniques. Stick to foods that are readily digestible, such as rice, bananas, and prepared vegetables, during a flare-up. Maintaining proper hydration, engaging in stress-reducing activities such as deep breathing exercises, and contemplating the use of over-the-counter remedies or prescribed medications to alleviate discomfort are all viable options.

VOLUME

CHAPTER FIVE

Commencing Your IBS Diet

It is crucial to identify your triggers by maintaining a food diary to begin managing IBS through diet. Monitor all of your food intake and document any symptoms to assist in identifying trends. Start with the low-FODMAP diet, which eliminates common IBS triggers such as certain fruits, vegetables, dairy, and wheat. Gradually reintroduce foods to determine which ones cause problems. Personalized guidance and nutritional balance can be achieved by consulting a dietitian.

Meal Planning

Balancing your diet with safe, low-FODMAP foods is essential for effective meal planning for IBS. Plan meals that consist of non-triggering vegetables, such as carrots, spinach, and bell peppers, and lean proteins, such as tofu or chicken. Incorporate soluble fibers, such as oats, into your diet and steer clear of high-fat, peppery, or oily foods that may exacerbate symptoms. Maintaining nutritional adequacy while managing IBS necessitates the development of a weekly menu that is both organized and diverse.

Tips For Shopping At The Grocery Store

Focus on fresh, whole foods and meticulously read labels when grocery shopping for an IBS-friendly diet. Select lactose-free dairy alternatives and opt for gluten-free cereals such as quinoa and rice. Processed foods that frequently contain high-FODMAP constituents, such as high fructose corn syrup or artificial sweeteners, should be avoided.

Shopping in the perimeter of the store, where fresh produce, meats, and dairy are stocked, can assist in avoiding processed and packaged products that may induce symptoms.

Batch Cooking And Meal Preparation

Managing IBS can be facilitated by preparing meals in advance. Cook large quantities of IBS-friendly dishes, such as quinoa salads, grilled chicken, or vegetable stews, and preserve them in individual servings. This guarantees that you have meals that are both safe and available to consume, which reduces the likelihood of consuming trigger foods when you are pressed for time. To facilitate adherence to your diet plan, refrigerate meals in hermetic containers for several days and freeze portions for extended storage.

Examining Food Labels

It is essential to read food labels to prevent the occurrence of IBS triggers. Select low-FODMAP ingredients and steer clear of high-FODMAP items, such as wheat, scallions, and garlic. Focus on the fiber content and serving sizes, with a preference for soluble fiber over insoluble fiber, which can exacerbate symptoms. Avoid foods that contain concealed carbohydrates and artificial sweeteners, including sorbitol and mannitol, as they may also induce IBS. Become acquainted with the most prevalent high-FODMAP constituents to make informed and convenient decisions during your purchasing trip.

Setting Realistic Goals

The effective management of IBS is facilitated by the establishment of realistic objectives. Begin by establishing modest, attainable goals, such as increasing one's water intake or incorporating a new IBS-friendly recipe every week.

Monitor your advancement and commemorate minor accomplishments to maintain your motivation. As you discover the foods that are most beneficial for you, be patient with yourself and modify your objectives as necessary. Remember, the management of IBS is a gradual process, and the implementation of consistent, modest adjustments can result in substantial improvements over time.

CHAPTER SIX

Your Diet And IBS

Diet is a critical factor in the management of Irritable Bowel Syndrome (IBS), as the dietary choices you make can have a substantial impact on your digestive health. Individuals with IBS frequently discover that certain foods exacerbate their symptoms, while others can assist in their relief. It is crucial to comprehend the extent to which your diet influences your condition, as a balanced diet that is customized to your requirements can assist in reducing the frequency and severity of IBS symptoms.

The Impact Of Diet On IBS Symptoms

The motility, sensitivity, and microbiome of the intestines are influenced by diet, which in turn impacts the symptoms of IBS. For example, diarrhea may result in certain individuals with IBS due to the increased motility of the intestines that high-fat and piquant foods can induce. In contrast, constipation may be the consequence of consuming low-fiber foods, which may impede digestion. Identifying and avoiding foods that elicit these symptoms is essential for the effective management of IBS, as what is effective for one individual may not be effective for another.

Examples Of Foods That Frequently Induce IBS

IBS symptoms are frequently precipitated by specific substances. Dairy products, legumes, caffeine, artificial sweeteners, certain fruits and vegetables (such as scallions and garlic), and high-fat foods are among the most prevalent perpetrators. For example, individuals with lactose intolerance may experience bloating and flatulence as a result of lactose in dairy products, a common occurrence in IBS. It is possible to mitigate the frequency and severity of IBS flare-ups by monitoring these triggers and modifying or eliminating them from one's diet.

Significance Of Individualized Dietary Plans

To effectively manage IBS, it is imperative to develop personalized dietary plans, as each person may have distinct tolerance levels and triggers. Work with a dietitian to identify specific foods that exacerbate your symptoms and to create a personalized dietary plan.

For instance, a low FODMAP diet may be advantageous for certain individuals, as it eliminates specific carbohydrates that are difficult to metabolize and can induce flatulence and bloating. Personalized plans guarantee that you can consume a diverse array of foods while simultaneously alleviating symptoms of IBS.

The Function Of Fiber In The Management Of IBS

The administration of IBS is influenced by the type and quantity of fiber, which can be either beneficial or problematic. Soluble fiber, which is present in foods such as apples and oats, is generally prescribed for individuals with IBS. It can assist in the regulation of digestive movements. Nevertheless, symptoms such as bloating and flatulence may be exacerbated by insoluble fiber, which is present in whole cereals and vegetables. By gradually increasing fiber intake and emphasizing soluble fiber, it is possible to more effectively manage symptoms of IBS.

Advantages Of Maintaining A Food Journal

Maintaining a food diary is a practical instrument for the management of IBS. You can identify patterns and isolate specific food triggers by documenting the food you consume, the timing of your meals, and any symptoms that may arise. For example, if you observe that symptoms worsen after consuming dairy or piquant foods, you can take measures to avoid these items. A food diary is a valuable tool for gaining a comprehensive understanding of the impact of your diet on your IBS. This information is essential for making informed dietary decisions and collaborating with healthcare providers to create an effective management plan.

High-FODMAP Foods Vs. Low-FODMAP Foods

In comparison to high-FODMAP foods, low-FODMAP foods are simpler to metabolize and less likely to induce IBS symptoms. For instance, bananas, blueberries, and strawberries are low-FODMAP fruits, whereas apples, pears, and mangoes are high-FODMAP fruits that can induce symptoms. In the same vein, low-FODMAP vegetables, including cucumbers, zucchini, and carrots, are preferred over high-FODMAP vegetables, including cauliflower, broccoli, and scallions. Regular milk and soft cheeses have high FODMAP, while lactose-free milk and firm cheeses have low FODMAP.

Advantages Of A Low-FODMAP Diet

A low-FODMAP diet can significantly reduce the symptoms of IBS, thereby enhancing the quality of life for those who are affected. Individuals frequently report reduced abdominal pain, flatulence, and bloating, as well as more consistent bowel movements, as a result of reducing their consumption of high-FODMAP foods.

This diet also aids in the identification of specific dietary triggers, thereby enabling a more personalized approach to the management of IBS.

Numerous individuals report experiencing increased energy and decreased anxiety regarding their digestive health as a result of adhering to a low-FODMAP diet.

Common Low-Fodmap Foods

Lean meats, eggs, fish, tofu, and lactose-free dairy products are among the most prevalent low-FODMAP foods. Fruits, including bananas, oranges, grapes, and kiwis, as well as vegetables like bell peppers, carrots, spinach, and tomatoes, are low in fructose monosaccharides (FODMAPs). Additionally, nuts and seeds such as almonds, peanuts, and chia seeds, as well as grains like rice, oatmeal, quinoa, and gluten-free bread, are considered safe options. These foods are the foundation of a low-FODMAP diet and can be combined to produce meals that are both balanced and satisfying.

Establishing A Low-FODMAP Pantry

The process of establishing a low-FODMAP larder entails the accumulation of appropriate foods and ingredients to facilitate the preparation of meals. Lactose-free milk, hard cheeses, and gluten-free cereals such as rice and quinoa are essential commodities.

It is advisable to maintain a supply of fresh low-FODMAP fruits and vegetables, as well as tinned versions that are devoid of high-FODMAP constituents. Additionally, it is advantageous to possess low-FODMAP munchies, including bland rice cakes, popcorn, and nuts. It is possible to effectively maintain a low-FODMAP diet by reading labels and ensuring that the pantry is devoid of high-FODMAP items.

CHAPTER SEVEN

Breakfast Recipes

Smoothie Bowls With Low FODMAP Content

Blend a tablespoon of chia seeds, half a banana, a fistful of strawberries, and a cup of lactose-free yogurt to create a low-FODMAP smoothie bowl. For a nutritious and gut-friendly start to your day, pour the smoothie into a bowl and garnish with sliced kiwi, a scattering of Low-FODMAP granola, and a few fresh blueberries.

Pancakes That Are Free Of Gluten

Mix one cup of gluten-free flour, one tablespoon of sugar, a teaspoon of baking powder, a sprinkle of salt, one egg, and one cup of lactose-free milk to make gluten-free pancakes. Cook the batter on a preheated griddle until bubbles appear on the surface and the margins appear set. Subsequently, rotate the batter and continue cooking until it turns golden brown. Serve with fresh fruit and pure maple syrup.

Granola With Low FODMAP Content

Combine rolled oats, shredded coconut, pumpkin seeds, and a drizzle of maple syrup to produce a low-FODMAP granola. Spread the mixture evenly on a baking sheet and bake at 325°F for 20 minutes, stirring halfway through. Once chilled, store in an airtight container and consume with lactose-free yogurt or a dash of almond milk.

Breakfast Options Based On Eggs

A straightforward vegetable omelet is an excellent option for a breakfast that is egg-based. Combine two eggs with a small amount of lactose-free milk, and then transfer the mixture to a non-stick skillet that is set over medium heat. Cook until the eggs are set and the vegetables are tender, then add diced bell peppers, parsley, and tomatoes.

Accompany the dish with avocado segments and a dash of salt and pepper.

Mix half a cup of lactose-free milk with half a cup of gluten-free cereals in a container to prepare overnight oats. Incorporate one tablespoon of chia seeds into the mixture and refrigerate it overnight. For a quick and substantial breakfast, simply top the oatmeal with sliced strawberries, a handful of blueberries, and a drizzle of maple syrup in the morning.

Lunch Recipes

It is imperative to prioritize meals that are mild on the digestive system when developing lunch options for individuals with Irritable Bowel Syndrome (IBS). Symptoms may be alleviated by selecting ingredients that are basic and readily digestible. Foods that are low in fermentable oligosaccharides, disaccharides, monosaccharides, and polyols (FODMAPs) should be included in lunch recipes, as they have the potential to exacerbate symptoms of IBS. A well-rounded supper can be achieved by incorporating a diverse selection of proteins, vegetables, and grains, all while minimizing discomfort. Here are a few supper recipe suggestions that are specifically designed for individuals with IBS.

Low-FODMAP Salads: Salads are adaptable and can be tailored to meet the dietary requirements and preferences of each individual. For those with IBS, it's crucial to select ingredients that are low in FODMAPs to prevent digestive discomfort. Choose verdant greens, such as spinach or kale, as a foundation and incorporate low-FODMAP vegetables, including carrots, bell peppers, and cucumbers. Consider incorporating grilled chicken, tofu, or hard-boiled eggs into the dish for protein. Dressings should be prepared using low-FODMAP constituents, such as vinegar, lemon juice, or olive oil. Onions, garlic, and croutons are high-FODMAP garnishes that should be avoided.

Rice and Quinoa Bowls: For those with IBS, rice and quinoa bowls are a nutritious and satisfying supper option. Rice and quinoa are both easily digestible and low in fructose-containing monosaccharides (FODMAPs), rendering them appropriate for individuals with sensitive stomachs.

Begin by incorporating a base of cooked rice or quinoa, followed by a protein source such as seared salmon, tofu, or turkey. For an increase in nutrients and flavor, incorporate low-FODMAP vegetables such as zucchini, spinach, and tomatoes. Add a layer of flavor by drizzling a low-FODMAP marinade or vinaigrette over the dish.

Low-FODMAP Soups: Soups can be a comforting and nourishing option for individuals with IBS, particularly during colder months or when experiencing digestive distress. Ingredients such as shallots, garlic, and high-FODMAP vegetables should be avoided when preparing low-FODMAP soups. Instead, choose a homemade bouillon or low-FODMAP stock as the foundation and incorporate protein sources such as chicken, tofu, or seafood.

Incorporate low-FODMAP vegetables, including spinach, green beans, and carrots, to enhance your nutritional intake. Season with herbs and seasonings that are well-tolerated, including ginger, oregano, and basil.

Sandwich and Wrap alternatives: Sandwiches and wraps are convenient lunch alternatives that can be readily customized to conform to a low-FODMAP diet.

When selecting bread or wraps, seek those that are prepared with low-FODMAP ingredients, such as maize tortillas or rice flour. Select protein sources such as sliced turkey, chicken, or tuna for the fillings.

Incorporate low-FODMAP vegetables, including cucumber, tomato, and lettuce, to enhance the flavor and texture of the dish. Exercise caution when selecting condiments, opting for low-FODMAP alternatives such as mayonnaise or mustard that do not contain high-FODMAP ingredients such as garlic or onion powder.

Dinner Recipes

With a few straightforward modifications, dinner can be both digestible and delectable for individuals with IBS. It is essential to choose low-FODMAP alternatives, such as grilled or roasted poultry or fish, which should be served with a side of steamed vegetables.

Experiment with flavorful herbs and seasonings that are mild on the stomach, such as ginger or basil, to improve the taste without eliciting symptoms. It is important to be mindful of portion sizes and to steer clear of common triggers, such as onions and garlic.

Low-FODMAP Pasta Dishes: Individuals with IBS do not have to refrain from consuming pasta. Seek out gluten-free alternatives that are simpler to digest, such as those derived from rice or quinoa.

For a substantial meal, add protein sources such as grilled shrimp or tofu and pair your pasta with a homemade low-FODMAP tomato sauce that is free of shallots and garlic. It is important to adhere to the recommended portion sizes to prevent your digestive system from being overloaded.

Grilled and Baked Protein Options: Adding variety to your diet by grilling or baking protein sources such as chicken, seafood, or tofu can be a flavorful and IBS-friendly option. Marinate your protein in basic, low-FODMAP ingredients, such as olive oil, lemon juice, and herbs like thyme or rosemary.

For a meal that is both digestible and well-balanced, consider serving it with a small side salad or a portion of steamed vegetables. This will not exacerbate symptoms of IBS.

Vegetable Stir-Fries: Prepare a nutritious and expeditious vegetable stir-fry for a supper that is both satisfying and gentle on the digestive system.

Opt for low-FODMAP vegetables, such as zucchini, carrots, and bell peppers, and steer clear of high-FODMAP options, such as onions and mushrooms. For an enhanced flavor without discomfort, incorporate a small quantity of low-FODMAP sauce, such as tamari or soy sauce, and season with ginger and garlic-infused oil.

Low-FODMAP Casseroles and Hearty Stews: Individuals with IBS can still relish warm, comforting casseroles and stews by selecting low-FODMAP ingredients and exercising portion control.

Select lean protein sources, such as turkey or lean beef, and robust vegetables, such as potatoes, carrots, and spinach. Utilize a low-FODMAP broth or sauce as a foundation and incorporate herbs and seasonings to improve flavor without inducing symptoms. To prevent symptoms, it is important to consume these dishes in moderation and regulate portion sizes.

CHAPTER EIGHT

Snacks And Desserts

Low-FODMAP refreshment suggestions: It is essential to select munchies that do not exacerbate symptoms when managing IBS. Instead, select snacks such as rice cakes with lactose-free cheese, carrot spears with hummus, or a scattering of almonds. These treats are low in fermentable carbohydrates (FODMAPs), which can exacerbate symptoms of IBS.

Healthy Low-FODMAP dessert recipes: These delectable low-FODMAP dessert recipes will satisfy your sugar appetite without causing any digestive distress. Consider preparing a delectable fruit salad featuring kiwi, blueberries, and strawberries, or indulging in a slice of lactose-free cheesecake with an almond flour crust.

These delicacies are mild on the digestive system and will not induce any discomfort.

Energy bites and bars: Prepare a quantity of low-FODMAP energy bites or bars for a fast and convenient refreshment on the go. For a delectable energy boost that will not induce symptoms of IBS, combine rolled oats, peanut butter, maple syrup, and dark chocolate morsels. These treats are an ideal choice for those who require an additional boost to maintain their energy levels during hectic days.

Low-FODMAP baking recipes: By employing low-FODMAP ingredients, you can indulge in domestic baked goods without experiencing digestive distress. Substitute wheat flour with gluten-free alternatives, such as rice flour or oat flour, and substitute conventional dairy with lactose-free milk or almond milk.

For a treat that is gentle on your digestion, consider creating a quantity of low-FODMAP banana muffins or chocolate chip cookies.

Smoothies and shakes: Begin your day with a nutritious and gut-friendly smoothie or shake. For a breakfast that is both low-FODMAP and delectable, combine spinach, banana, lactose-free yogurt, and a few strawberries in a blender. In addition, you may incorporate a teaspoon of protein powder to provide an additional energy boost. Smoothies and smoothies are a convenient method of consuming nutrients while avoiding problematic FODMAPs.

Smoothies And Beverages

It is crucial to select low-FODMAP beverages for the treatment of IBS. Water, herbal teas, and specific fruit concoctions are among the beverages that should be consumed in moderation. It is possible to prevent the onset of symptoms by refraining from consuming high-FODMAP beverages, such as certain fruit juices, carbonated beverages, and alcohol. Smoothies can be an effective method for incorporating nutrients while managing IBS. Choose low-FODMAP ingredients, such as bananas, spinach, and lactose-free yogurt.

Exercise caution when consuming fruits that are high in fructose (FODMAPs), such as apples and mangoes. A soothing and invigorating alternative for individuals with sensitive stomachs can be achieved by combining these ingredients with water or lactose-free milk.

Low-Fodmap Beverage Alternatives

Minimizing digestive distress is imperative for individuals with IBS, and low-FODMAP drink options are essential. Although water is the optimal choice, lactose-free milk, almond milk, and coconut water are also viable alternatives. It is recommended that fruit juices be ingested in moderation and from low-FODMAP fruits, such as citrus fruits and berries. It is essential to refrain from consuming high-FODMAP beverages, including carbonated beverages, certain fruit juices, and beverages that contain artificial sweeteners, to prevent the exacerbation of symptoms. Selecting beverages that are appropriate for one's preferences necessitates reading labels and considering serving quantities.

Digestion-Enhancing Herbal Teas

Those with IBS may find herbal infusions to be calming, as they provide relief from digestive discomfort. Peppermint tea is particularly advantageous for alleviating symptoms such as flatulence and bloating and soothing the digestive tract. Ginger tea has the potential to improve digestion and mitigate nausea. Chamomile tea is recognized for its tranquil properties, which may alleviate stress-related symptoms of IBS. Opt for botanical teas that are in their purest form, devoid of artificial flavors or added carbohydrates. The consumption of botanical infusions between meals can facilitate relaxation and enhance the overall health of the digestive system.

Smoothie Recipes With Low-FODMAP Content

While assuring appropriate nutrition, the creation of low-FODMAP smoothies can be a delectable method of managing IBS symptoms. Adding a small quantity of almond milk, spinach, banana, and lactose-free yogurt to a blender is a straightforward recipe. Protein and fiber content can be enhanced without exacerbating symptoms by incorporating a spoonful of peanut butter or a scattering of chia seeds. Refrain from consuming high-FODMAP constituents, such as honey, pears, and apples. By experimenting with various combinations of low-FODMAP fruits and lactose-free liquids, it is possible to develop customized smoothie recipes that are mild on the digestive system.

IBS Hydration Tips

It is essential to maintain proper hydration for the well-being of all individuals, particularly those who have IBS. A prevalent symptom of IBS is constipation, which can be prevented by drinking water throughout the day to sustain proper digestion.

Carry a reusable water container and consume water regularly to guarantee sufficient hydration. Hydration can also be facilitated by herbal infusions, coconut water, and low-FODMAP fruit-infused water. It is crucial to refrain from consuming an excessive amount of caffeine and alcohol, as both can exacerbate IBS symptoms and dehydrate the body.

Monitoring urine color can function as a straightforward indicator of hydration status, to achieve a delicate yellow hue. Hydration levels can also be maintained by incorporating hydrating foods such as cucumber, watermelon, and citrus into meals and snacks.

CHAPTER NINE

Seven Days Meal Plan, Recipes, Ingredients, And Detailed Preparatory Guidelines For Irritable Bowel Syndrome

DAY ONE:

Breakfast: Banana Smoothie Bowl

- **INGREDIENTS**:

o One mature banana

o 1/2 cup of lactose-free yogurt

o 1/2 cup of almond milk

o One tablespoon of chia seeds

O 1/4 cup of blueberries

o 1/4 cup of cut strawberries

o One tablespoon of almond butter

• *PREPARATION:*

1. Blend the almond milk, lactose-free yogurt, and banana until they are completely smooth.

2. Transfer the mixture to a vessel and garnish with almond butter, blueberries, strawberries, and chia seeds.

Lunch: Quinoa and Roasted Vegetable Salad

• **INGREDIENTS**:

o One cup of prepared quinoa

o One zucchini, minced

o One minced bell pepper

o. Half a cup of cherry tomatoes

o 1/4 cup of finely minced herbs

o Two tablespoons of olive oil

o Add salt and pepper to taste

• *PREPARATION:*

1. Preheat the oven to 400°F (200°C).

2. Combine zucchini and bell pepper with olive oil, salt, and pepper.

3. Roast for 20 minutes.

4. Combine quinoa, cherry tomatoes, and parsley with roasted vegetables.

Dinner: Baked Salmon with Steamed Asparagus

• **INGREDIENTS**:

o One salmon tenderloin

o One bundle of asparagus, trimmed

o One tablespoon of olive oil

o One citrus

o Add salt and pepper to taste

• *PREPARATION:*

1. Preheat the oven to 375°F (190°C).

2. Drizzle olive oil, salt, and pepper over the salmon and place it on a baking sheet.

3. Bake for 20-25 minutes.

4. Steam asparagus for 5-7 minutes and serve with salmon and a lemon wedge.

Snack: Rice Cakes with Almond Butter

• **INGREDIENTS**:

o Two rice dumplings

o Two tablespoons of almond butter

Carrot Ginger Juice

• **INGREDIENTS**:

o Four vegetables

o One-inch slice of ginger

o One apple

• *PREPARATION:*

1. Combine the carrots, ginger, and apple into a single juice.

DAY TWO:

Breakfast: Oatmeal with Berries

• **INGREDIENTS**:

o 1/2 cup of dried oats

o One cup of almond milk or water

O 1/4 cup of blueberries

O 1/4 cup of raspberries

• One tablespoon of maple syrup

• PREPARATION:

1. Follow the instructions on the package when cooking cereals with water or almond milk.

2. Add berries to the top and drizzle with maple syrup.

Lunch: Spinach Salad and Grilled Chicken

• **INGREDIENTS**:

o One roasted chicken breast, divided

o Two bowls of young spinach

o 1/4 cup of cut strawberries

o One-quarter avocado, diced

o Two tablespoons of balsamic vinaigrette

1. Arrange spinach on a platter.

2. Garnish with seared chicken, strawberries, and avocado, and drizzle with vinaigrette.

Dinner: Zucchini Noodles with Turkey Meatballs

INGREDIENTS

o One pound of minced poultry

o One egg

1/4 cup of breadcrumbs without gluten

o One teaspoon of dried oregano

o Two spiralized zucchinis

o One cup of marinara sauce

• *PREPARATION:*

1. Preheat the oven to 375°F (190°C).

2. Combine turkey, egg, breadcrumbs, and oregano. Shape the mixture into meatballs.

3. Bake for 20 minutes.

4. Toss zucchini linguine with warm marinara sauce.

5. Serve the meatballs with zucchini linguine.

Snack: Hummus with carrot sticks

• **INGREDIENTS**:

o One cup of carrot spears

o 1/4 cup of hummus

Apple and Spinach Juice

• **INGREDIENTS**:

o One cup of spinach

o Two peaches

o One cucumber

• *PREPARATION:*

1. Combine the spinach, apples, and cucumber in a juicer.

THIRD DAY:

Breakfast: Chia Seed Pudding

• **INGREDIENTS**:

o Three teaspoons of chia seeds

o One cup of almond milk

• One tablespoon of maple syrup

O 1/4 cup of raspberries

• PREPARATION:

1. Combine almond milk, maple syrup, and chia seeds.

2. Place in the refrigerator for the night.

3. Before serving, top with blackberries.

Lunch: Lentil Soup

• INGREDIENTS:

o One cup of lentils

o One carrot, diced

o One celery stalk, minced

o One minced onion

o Four pints of vegetable broth

o One teaspoon of cardamom

o Add salt and pepper to taste

• PREPARATION:

1. Sauté the carrot, celery, and onion until they are tender.

2. Cumin, bouillon, and lentils should be incorporated.

3. Allow the legumes to simmer for 30 minutes until they are soft.

Dinner: Shrimp Stir-Fry with Rice

INGREDIENTS

o One cup of shrimp, skinned and deveined

o One sliced bell pepper

o One zucchini, cut

o Two tablespoons of olive oil

o One cup of prepared rice

o Add salt and pepper to taste

• *PREPARATION:*

1. Heat olive oil in a pan and sauté shrimp until they are golden.

2. Add zucchini and bell pepper; sauté until they are soft.

3. Serve with couscous.

Snack: Blueberry Almond Mix

• **INGREDIENTS**:

O 1/4 cup of blueberries

o 1/4 cup of almonds

Orange-carrot juice

• **INGREDIENTS**:

o Two peaches

o Two vegetables

· *PREPARATION*.

1. Combine the juices of the citrus and vegetables.

DAY FOUR:

Smoothie for breakfast

· INGREDIENTS:

o One banana

o 1/2 cup of spinach

o 1/2 cup of almond milk

o One tablespoon of flaxseed

· *PREPARATION:*

1. All ingredients should be blended until they are

homogeneous.

INGREDIENTS

o One cup of prepared legumes

o One diced cucumber

o 1/4 cup cherry tomatoes, halved

o Two tablespoons of olive oil

o One tablespoon of lemon juice

o Add salt and pepper to taste

• *PREPARATION:*

1. Combine tomatoes, cucumbers, and legumes.

2. Season with salt, pepper, lemon juice, and olive oil.

• **INGREDIENTS**:

o One halibut fillet

o One tablespoon of olive oil

o One citrus

o One cup of green beans, trimmed

o Add salt and pepper to taste

• *PREPARATION:*

1. Preheat the oven to 375°F (190°C).

2. Place the cod on a baking sheet and drizzle with olive oil, salt, and pepper.

3. Bake for 20-25 minutes.

4. Serve cod with a wedge of lemon and steamed green beans.

Snack: Rice Cakes with Sliced Avocado

INGREDIENTS

o Two rice dumplings

o One-quarter avocado, diced

Juice: Green Juice

• **INGREDIENTS**:

o One cup of spinach

o One cucumber

o One apple

• *PREPARATION:*

1. Combine the spinach, cucumber, and apple in a juicer.

DAY FIVE:

Breakfast: Oatmeal that has been prepared overnight

• **INGREDIENTS**:

o 1/2 cup of dried oats

o 1/2 cup of almond milk

o One tablespoon of chia seeds

• One tablespoon of maple syrup

O 1/4 cup of blueberries

• *PREPARATION:*

1. Combine almond milk, chia seeds, maple syrup, and cereals.

2. Place in the refrigerator for the night.

3. Before serving, sprinkle blueberries on top.

• INGREDIENTS:

o One gluten-free tortilla

o 1/4 avocado, pureed

o One-quarter cup of shredded lettuce

o 1/4 cup of grated carrot

o Three slices of turkey breast

• *PREPARATION:*

1. Apply pureed avocado to a tortilla.

2. Layer turkey, carrots, and lettuce.

3. Roll up and serve.

Dinner: Sweet Potatoes and Grilled Chicken

• INGREDIENTS:

o One chicken breast

o One sweet potato, divided

o One tablespoon of olive oil

o One teaspoon of rosemary

o Add salt and pepper to taste

• *PREPARATION:*

1. Preheat the barbecue and broil the chicken until it is fully cooked.

2. Combine rosemary, olive oil, salt, and pepper with the sweet potato.

3. Preheat the oven to 400°F (200°C) and bake for 25-30 minutes.

4. Serve poultry with sweet potato.

Snack: Hummus with Cucumber Slices

• **INGREDIENTS**:

o One cup of cucumber segments

o 1/4 cup of hummus

• **INGREDIENTS**:

o Two beets

o Two vegetables

o One apple

• *PREPARATION:*

1. Combine the beets, carrots, and apples in a juicer.

DAY SIX:

Breakfast: Yogurt Parfait

• **INGREDIENTS**:

o 1/2 cup of lactose-free yogurt

o 1/4 cup of gluten-free granola

o 1/4 cup of assorted fruit

• PREPARATION:

1. Arrange yogurt, granola, and berries in a glass.

Lunch: Quinoa and Spinach Salad

• INGREDIENTS:

o One cup of prepared quinoa

o Two bowls of young spinach

o 1/4 cup of sliced walnuts

o One-quarter cup of dried cranberries

o Two tablespoons of balsamic vinaigrette

• PREPARATION:

1. Combine cranberries, almonds, spinach, and quinoa.

2. Use a balsamic vinaigrette to dress.

• **INGREDIENTS**:

o Two bell peppers

o One cup of prepared quinoa

o 1/2 cup of black legumes

o 1/2 cup of maize

o One-quarter cup of salsa

• *PREPARATION:*

1. Turn the oven on to 375°F, or 190°C.

2. Remove the seeds and cut the heads off the peppers.

3. Combine salsa, maize, black beans, and quinoa.

4. Fill peppers with the mixture.

5. Bake for a duration of 30-35 minutes.

Snack: Almond butter on apple slices

INGREDIENTS

o One apple, cut

o Two tablespoons of almond butter

Pineapple Mint Juice: Juice

• **INGREDIENTS**:

o 1/2 pineapple

o One fistful of mint fronds

• *PREPARATION:*

1. Combine the pineapple and mint juices.

SEVENTH DAY:

Breakfast: Pancakes with bananas

• **INGREDIENTS**:

o One banana

o Two eggs

o One-quarter teaspoon of baking powder

o One-quarter teaspoon of cinnamon

• PREPARATION:

1. Combine eggs, baking powder, and cinnamon with the mashed banana.

2. Cook in a non-stick pan until it turns golden brown.

Lunch: Chicken and Avocado Salad

• INGREDIENTS:

o One roasted chicken breast, divided

o One minced avocado

o 1/4 cup cherry tomatoes, halved

o Two bowls of assorted greens

o Two tablespoons of olive oil

o One tablespoon of lemon juice

• *PREPARATION:*

1. Combine chicken, avocado, tomatoes, and vegetables.

2. Use olive oil and lemon juice to dress.

Dinner: Brown Rice with Baked Tilapia

• **INGREDIENTS**:

o One fillet of tilapia

o One cup of brown rice that has been prepared

o One tablespoon of olive oil

o One citrus

o Add salt and pepper to taste

- *PREPARATION:*

1. Turn the oven on to 375°F, or 190°C.

2. Place the tilapia on a baking sheet and season with salt, pepper, and olive oil.

3. Bake for 20 minutes.

4. Serve with brown rice and a wedge of lemon.

Snack: A Variety of Nuts

- **INGREDIENTS**:

o 1/4 cup of assorted nuts (walnuts, cashews, almonds)

Juice: Cucumber-Lemon Juice

- **INGREDIENTS**:

o One cucumber

o One citrus

1. Combine the cucumber and lemon juice.

The following seven-day meal plan for IBS offers a diverse selection of meals that are mild on the digestive system, with an emphasis on low-FODMAP foods whenever feasible. The recipes are intended to be both nutritious and simple to prepare, thereby promoting a balanced diet and alleviating symptoms of IBS.

CHAPTER TEN

Seven Desserts Procedural Recipes For Irritable Bowel Syndrome (IBS) Diet And Guidelines

Irritable bowel syndrome (IBS) is a prevalent gastrointestinal disorder that can be effectively managed by adjusting one's diet. This article contains seven confection recipes that are suitable for individuals with IBS and are mild on the digestive system.

1. BANANA-OAT COOKIES

INGREDIENTS:

• Two mature avocados

• One cup of gluten-free toasted oats

• 1/4 cup of dairy-free dark chocolate chunks

STEPS:

1. Set the oven's temperature to 175°C/350°F.

2. In a basin, mash the bananas until they are pureed.

3. Incorporate the rolled oats until they are thoroughly mixed.

4. Incorporate the chocolate morsels by folding them in.

5. Drop spoonfuls of the mixture onto a baking sheet that has been lined with parchment paper.

6. Bake for 15 minutes or until the surface is a rich golden color.

7. Before serving, let it cool.

Guidelines: These pastries are abundant in fiber from bananas and oats, which promotes digestion without irritating the gastrointestinal tract.

INGREDIENTS:

• One cup of dairy-free coconut yogurt

• One-half cup of organic blueberries

• One tablespoon of chia seeds

STEPS:

1. Spoon the coconut yogurt into a dish.

2. Add a layer of fresh blueberries on top.

3. Sprinkle chia seeds on top.

4. Gently stir and allow the chia seeds to soften for five minutes.

Guidelines: Blueberries are a source of fiber and antioxidants, while coconut yogurt is an excellent substitute for individuals who steer clear of dairy.

INGREDIENTS:

• One cup of strained almond milk

• Three tablespoons of chia seeds

• One tablespoon of maple syrup (optional)

• 1/2 teaspoon of vanilla extract

STEPS:

1. Combine the almond milk, chia seeds, maple syrup, and vanilla extract in a bowl or jar.

2. Combine thoroughly.

3. Stir occasionally to prevent clumping, and refrigerate for a minimum of four hours or overnight.

4. Chill before serving.

Guidelines: Chia seeds are highly beneficial for digestion and offer a smooth, milky texture that is suitable for individuals with sensitive stomachs.

4. APPLE CINNAMON COMPOTE

INGREDIENTS:

• Two apples (peeled, cored, and minced)

• 1/2 teaspoon of dried cinnamon

• One tablespoon of maple syrup

• 1/4 cup water

STEPS:

1. Combine apples, cinnamon, maple syrup, and water in a saucepan over medium heat.

2. Cook, stirring occasionally, until apples are tender, about 10-15 minutes.

3. Before serving, remove from the flame and allow to cool slightly.

Guidelines: Apples are an excellent source of pectin and fiber, which can help regulate bowel movements.

5. RICE PUDDING

INGREDIENTS:

• One-half cup of white rice

• 2 cups of strained almond milk

• 1/4 cup of maple syrup

• 1/2 teaspoon of dried cinnamon

STEPS:

1. Thoroughly rinse the rice with cool water.

2. In a saucepan over medium heat, combine almond milk and rice.

3. After bringing the mixture to a boil, lower the heat and simmer it while stirring. frequently, until the rice is tender and the mixture is velvety, which should take approximately 20-25 minutes.

4. Add the maple syrup and cinnamon to the mixture.

5. Let it cool down a little before serving.

Guidelines: This confection is complemented by a comforting, easily digestible base of white rice, which is mild on the digestive system.

6. KIWI SORBET

INGREDIENTS:

• Four mature kiwis, peeled and sliced

• Two tablespoons of honey (or maple syrup for a vegan option)

• 1/4 cup of water

STEPS:

1. In a blender, combine the water, honey, and kiwis until the mixture is homogeneous.

2. Transfer the mixture to a shallow container and freeze for a minimum of four hours. Stir the mixture every hour to dislodge ice crystals.

3. Transfer the mixture to dishes and serve.

Guidelines: Kiwi is a revitalizing option for individuals with IBS and contains actinidin, an enzyme that aids digestion.

7. BROWNIES MADE WITH ALMOND FLOUR

INGREDIENTS:

• One cup of almond flour

• 1/4 cup of cocoa powder

• One-half cup of maple syrup

• 1/4 cup of heated coconut oil

• Two eggs (or flax eggs for a vegan option)

• One teaspoon of vanilla extract

• 1/2 teaspoon of baking powder

STEPS:

1. Set the oven's temperature to 175°C/350°F.

2. Combine almond flour, cocoa powder, and baking powder in a basin.

3. Whisk together maple syrup, coconut oil, eggs, and vanilla extract in a separate basin.

4. Stir the moist and dry ingredients until they are thoroughly combined.

5. Transfer the batter to a baking pan that has been greased.

6. Bake for 20-25 minutes or until a toothpick inserted into the center comes out clean.

7. Allow the mixture to settle before slicing it into squares.

Almond flour is a gluten-free, low-carb alternative that is more easily digestible than traditional wheat flour.

IBS-Friendly Dessert Guidelines

1. Low FODMAP Ingredients: Emphasize ingredients that are low in fermentable oligosaccharides, disaccharides, monosaccharides, and polyols.

2. Gluten-Free Alternatives: Numerous individuals with IBS experience alleviation by refraining from consuming gluten.

3. Dairy Alternatives: To prevent symptoms from arising, consume lactose-free or dairy-free products, such as almond or coconut milk.

4. Natural Sweeteners: In moderation, choose natural sweeteners such as maple syrup or honey, and refrain from consuming high fructose corn syrup.

5. Avoid Artificial Sweeteners and Additives: IBS symptoms may be exacerbated by artificial sweeteners and additives.

6. Portion Control: The consumption of smaller portions can assist in the prevention of digestive system excess.

7. Monitor Fiber Consumption: Maintain a balance between soluble and insoluble fiber to prevent the exacerbation of symptoms.

Individuals with IBS can indulge in delectable delicacies without jeopardizing their digestive health by adhering to these guidelines and incorporating these recipes.

CHAPTER ELEVEN

Seven Smoothies Procedural Recipes For Irritable Bowel Syndrome And Guidelines

Irritable Bowel Syndrome (IBS) is a prevalent gastrointestinal disorder that impacts the large intestine, resulting in symptoms such as abdominal pain, bloating, flatulence, diarrhea, or constipation.

Smoothies can be a nutritious and calming alternative when managing IBS, which frequently necessitates dietary modifications. The following are seven smoothie recipes that are suitable for individuals with IBS, as well as some recommendations to assist in the effective management of symptoms.

Smoothies that are suitable for individuals with IBS should adhere to the following guidelines:

1. Low-FODMAP Ingredients: Opt for fruits and vegetables that are low in fermentable oligosaccharides, disaccharides, monosaccharides, and polyols (FODMAPs), as these can exacerbate symptoms of IBS.

2. Refrain from Consuming High-Fat Ingredients: IBS symptoms may be exacerbated by high-fat foods. Therefore, it is advisable to consume low-fat yogurt, milk, or dairy alternatives.

3. Soluble fiber can assist in the management of IBS symptoms by modulating bowel movements. Oats, avocados, and flaxseeds are all viable sources.

4. Moderate Portions: To prevent symptoms from arising, it is recommended that smoothie servings be limited to approximately 8-10 ounces.

5. Maintain Hydration: To minimize sugar intake and maintain hydration, substitute fruit juices with water, ice, or medicinal beverages as a base.

6. Fresh and Natural: Choose fruits and vegetables that are either fresh or frozen and do not contain any added carbohydrates or preservatives.

7. Steer clear of artificial sweeteners: IBS symptoms may be precipitated by artificial sweeteners, particularly sorbitol and mannitol.

1. BLUEBERRY BANANA BLISS

INGREDIENTS:

• One mature banana

• ½ cup of blueberries, either fresh or preserved

• One cup of almond milk that is lactose-free

• One tablespoon of chia seeds

• ½ teaspoon of vanilla extract

STEPS:

1. Slice the banana after it has been peeled.

2. Add the banana, blueberries, almond milk, chia seeds, and vanilla extract to a blender.

3. Blend until the mixture is velvety and smooth.

4. Pour the beverage into a glass and savor it immediately.

2. STRAWBERRY SPINACH SMOOTHIE

INGREDIENTS:

• One cup of freshly hulled strawberries

• One fistful of young spinach

- One cup of lactose-free coconut milk

- One tablespoon of flaxseeds

- One teaspoon of maple syrup (optional)

STEPS:

1. Thoroughly rinse the spinach and strawberries.

2. In a blender, combine coconut milk, flaxseeds, maple syrup, strawberries, and greens.

3. Blend until the mixture is well-integrated and homogeneous.

4. Chill before serving.

3. TROPICAL DELIGHT

INGREDIENTS:

- One cup of diced pineapple

- One small, mature banana

- One cup of lactose-free yogurt

- ½ cup of ice or water

- One teaspoon of minced ginger

STEPS:

1. Slice the banana and dice the pineapple.

2. Blend the pineapple, banana, yogurt, water or ice, and ginger in the blender.

3. Blend until the mixture is frothy and smooth.

4. Pour the mixture into a glass and serve it immediately.

4. GREEN SMOOTHIE FOR RELAXATION

INGREDIENTS:

- One sliced and peeled kiwi

- One small cucumber, peeled and sliced

- One fistful of young spinach

- One cup of almond milk that is lactose-free

- One tablespoon of chia seeds

STEPS:

1. Slice the cucumber and kiwi.

2. Add the chia seeds, almond milk, spinach, cucumber, and kiwi to the blender.

3. Blend until the mixture is velvety and smooth.

4. For optimal outcomes, serve immediately.

5. SMOOTHIE WITH PAPAYA FLAVOR

INGREDIENTS:

- 1 cup of diced, peeled, and ripe papaya

- One small, mature banana

- One cup of lactose-free yogurt

• One tablespoon of honey (optional)

• ½ cup of ice or water

STEPS:

1. Dice the papaya and peel it.

2. Add yogurt, honey, banana, papaya, and water or ice to the blender.

3. Blend until the mixture is thick and smooth.

4. Pour the beverage into a glass and savor it.

6. MANGO AND CARROT SMOOTHIE

INGREDIENTS:

• One medium carrot, peeled and chopped

• One cup of diced mango

• One cup of lactose-free coconut milk

• One tablespoon of flaxseeds

• ½ teaspoon of turmeric powder

STEPS:

1. Chop and peel the carrot.

2. Combine the carrot, mango, coconut milk, flaxseeds, and turmeric in the blender.

3. Blend until the mixture is velvety and smooth.

4. Immediately serve as a delightfully refreshing treat.

7. SMOOTHIE WITH MELON AND MINT

INGREDIENTS:

• Diced 1 cup of honeydew melon or cantaloupe

• One handful of fresh mint leaves

• One cup of almond milk that is lactose-free

• One tablespoon of chia seeds

• ½ cup of ice or water

STEPS:

1. Cut the melon into small pieces.

2. Add the chia seeds, almond milk, water or ice, mint leaves, and melon to the blender.

3. Blend until the mixture is well-integrated and homogeneous.

4. Chill before serving.

These seven smoothies are designed to be mild on the digestive system while providing essential nutrients and hydration.

By following the guidelines and using the suggested ingredients, individuals with IBS can enjoy delectable and soothing smoothies without aggravating their symptoms. Always remember to consult with a healthcare provider before making significant dietary adjustments, particularly if you have a medical condition like IBS.

Meal Planning And Tips For Success

Meal planning is crucial for managing irritable bowel syndrome (IBS) symptoms. Begin by constructing a weekly meal plan that includes a variety of low-FODMAP foods such as lean proteins, fruits, vegetables, and grains. To save time during the week, consider bulk preparing and freezing dishes.

For example, you can prepare a large quantity of low-FODMAP chili or soup and divide it into individual servings to freeze for later use. When eating out, investigate restaurants in advance to discover options that align with your dietary requirements. It's also essential to communicate your dietary restrictions to the waitstaff to ensure your meal is prepared accordingly.

In social situations, don't hesitate to bring your low-FODMAP dish or munchies to ensure you have something safe to consume. Lastly, maintaining digestive health in the long term involves remaining consistent with your low-FODMAP diet, staying hydrated, managing stress, and getting regular exercise.

This approach to meal planning simplifies the process of adhering to a low-FODMAP diet by providing practical strategies for success in various situations. By incorporating batch cooking, researching restaurant options, and advocating for your dietary needs in social settings, managing IBS becomes more manageable.

Additionally, concentrating on long-term maintenance ensures ongoing digestive health.

Conclusion

The conclusion on the irritable bowel syndrome (IBS) diet underscores the significance of personalized dietary management to alleviate symptoms and enhance the quality of life for IBS sufferers. A one-size-fits-all approach is ineffectual due to the variability in individual stimuli and responses. However, certain dietary strategies have shown consistent benefits across many patients. The low FODMAP diet, which entails limiting intake of fermentable oligosaccharides, disaccharides, monosaccharides, and polyols, has been particularly effective in managing IBS symptoms such as bloating, gas, and abdominal pain. Additionally, identifying and avoiding specific food intolerances through an elimination diet can also be beneficial.

Moreover, incorporating high-fiber foods, remaining hydrated, and consuming regular, balanced meals can promote digestive health. Probiotics may offer symptom alleviation for some individuals by balancing gastrointestinal microbiota. IBS patients must work with healthcare professionals, including dietitians, to develop a tailored diet plan that considers their unique symptoms and nutritional requirements.

Ultimately, while dietary modifications can substantially reduce IBS symptoms, ongoing research is essential to further understand the condition and refine dietary recommendations. Patient education and support play a vital role in the successful management of IBS, empowering individuals to make informed dietary choices and enhance their overall well-being.

THE END